The Model

A Motivational Book

Dr. Monique Rodgers

The Model: A Motivational Book

Dr. Monique Rodgers

Called To Intercede Volume 13

Praying for Churches

Dr. Monique Rodgers

United States of America

Published by Shooting Stars Publishing House 2023
Copyright © 2023 Dr. Monique Rodgers

All Rights Reserved.

ISBN:9798397419413

This book has been published with all reasonable efforts taken to make the material error-free after the consent of the author. No part of this book shall be used, reproduced in any manner whatsoever without written permission from the author, except in the case of brief quotations embodied in critical articles and reviews.

The Author of this book is solely responsible and liable for its content including but not limited to the views, representations, descriptions, statements, information, opinions, and references. The Content of this book shall not constitute or be construed or deemed to reflect the opinion or expression of the Publisher or Editor. Neither the Publisher nor Editor endorse or approve the Content of this book or guarantee the reliability, accuracy or completeness of the Content published herein and do not make any representations or warranties of any kind, express or implied, including but not limited to the implied warranties of merchantability, fitness for a particular purpose. The Publisher and Editor shall not be liable whatsoever for any errors, omissions, whether such errors or omissions result from negligence, accident, or any other cause or claims for loss or damages of any kind, including without limitation, indirect or consequential loss or damage arising out of use, inability to use, or about the reliability, accuracy or sufficiency of the information contained in this book.

The Model: A Motivational Book

Dr. Monique Rodgers

DEDICATION

This book is dedicated to the models of the world.

Called To Intercede Volume 13

Praying for Churches

Dr. Monique Rodgers

Contents

Dedication……………………………………….

Introduction……………………………………..

Chapter One…………………………………….

Chapter Two……………………………………

Chapter Three…………………………………..

Chapter Four……………………………………

Chapter Five……………………………………

Chapter Six……………………………………

Affirmations for models……………………….

Fashion tips for models………………………..

Called To Intercede Volume 13

Praying for Churches

Dr. Monique Rodgers

Introduction

Modeling, an art form that has captivated the world for centuries, is a profession that embodies beauty, elegance, and self-expression. From the iconic supermodels who graced the covers of magazines to the aspiring talents who walk the runways of high-fashion events, the world of modeling has always held a certain allure. It is a realm where style, creativity, and determination converge, requiring hard work, dedication, and a passion for fashion.

In this comprehensive guide, we invite you to embark on a journey into the captivating world of modeling. Whether you dream of strutting your stuff on the catwalks of Paris, gracing the glossy pages of fashion magazines, or becoming the face of renowned brands, this book will equip you with the tools and knowledge you need to succeed in this highly competitive industry.

We will unravel the intricate tapestry of the modeling world, offering insights and practical advice that will empower you to navigate its challenges and seize its opportunities. From runway shows to photo shoots, casting calls to building your portfolio, we will cover every essential aspect of the modeling profession. Our aim is to provide you with a comprehensive understanding of the industry, empowering you to make informed decisions and embark on a successful modeling career.

Within these pages, you will discover the secrets of walking the runway with confidence and grace, mastering the art of posing for the camera, and developing your unique personal brand. We will delve into the business side of modeling, exploring contract negotiations, networking strategies, and the importance of self-promotion. Moreover, we will address the physical and emotional well-being of models, highlighting the significance of self-care, body positivity, and maintaining a balanced lifestyle.

Throughout this journey, we will draw upon the wisdom and experiences of industry professionals, top models, photographers, and fashion insiders. Their insights will provide invaluable guidance as you navigate the multifaceted world of modeling, learning from their successes, and gaining a deeper understanding of the industry's dynamics.

Whether you are an aspiring model taking your first steps or a seasoned professional seeking to refine your craft, this book is designed to be your trusted companion. Its pages are filled with practical advice, inspiring stories, and expert tips that will help you unlock your full potential as a model and set yourself apart in this ever-evolving industry.

So, are you ready to embrace the art and business of modeling? Let us embark on this exhilarating journey together, exploring the depths of your talent, igniting your passion for fashion, and equipping you with the tools you need to thrive. Whether your dreams lie in the lights of the runway or the allure of the fashion editorial, this book will serve as your guide, empowering you to pursue your aspirations and make your mark in the captivating world of modeling.

.

Chapter 1:
The Basics of Modeling

In this chapter, we will cover the basics of modeling, including the different types of modeling, the requirements for becoming a model, and the skills you need to succeed in the industry. We will also discuss the importance of networking and building relationships in the fashion industry.

Modeling is a profession that requires a combination of natural talent, hard work, and dedication. It is a highly competitive industry, and to succeed, you need to have a good understanding of the basics of modeling. In this chapter, we will cover the different types of modeling, the requirements for becoming a model, and the skills you need to succeed in the industry.

Types of Modeling:

There are several different types of modeling, and each requires a different set of skills and attributes. The most common types of modeling include:

1. **Fashion Modeling**: This is the most well-known type of modeling and involves modeling clothing and accessories for fashion designers and brands.

2. **Commercial Modeling**: This type of modeling involves modeling for advertisements, catalogs, and other commercial purposes.

3. **Fitness Modeling**: This type of modeling involves modeling for fitness brands and magazines and requires a fit and toned physique.

4. **Glamour Modeling**: This type of modeling involves modeling for men's magazines and requires a sultry and seductive look.

Requirements for Becoming a Model:

To become a model, there are several requirements you need to meet. These include:

1. Height: For fashion modeling, you need to be at least 5'8" for women and 6'0" for men. For commercial modeling, there is no height requirement.

2. Age: Most models start their careers in their late teens or early twenties, but there is no age limit for modeling.

3. Body Type: For fashion modeling, you need to have a slim and toned physique. For commercial modeling, there is no specific body type requirement.

4. **Skin and Hair**: Models need to have clear skin and healthy hair.

Skills for Modeling:

To succeed in the modeling industry, you need to have a combination of natural talent and learned skills. Some of the essential skills for modeling include:

1. **Posing**: Models need to know how to pose for the camera and how to move their bodies to create the desired effect.

2. **Facial Expressions:** Models need to know how to convey different emotions with their facial expressions.

3. **Confidence**: Models need to be confident in themselves and their abilities.

4. **Professionalism:** Models need to be professional and

reliable, showing up on time and ready to work.

5. **Communication:** Models need to be able to communicate effectively with photographers, designers, and other industry professionals.

Called To Intercede Volume 13

Praying for Churches

Dr. Monique Rodgers

The world of modeling is so very exciting! In this chapter, we will lay the groundwork for your modeling journey by exploring the essential basics that form the foundation of a successful modeling career. From understanding the different types of modeling to developing your unique look and style, we will delve into the fundamental aspects that will set you on the path to success.

1.1 The Many Faces of Modeling

Modeling is a diverse field with various avenues for exploration. Understanding the different types of modeling will help you identify where your interests and strengths lie. From high fashion and runway modeling to commercial, editorial, plus-size, and fitness modeling, each branch has its own unique requirements and opportunities. We will explore the distinctions between these areas and help you determine which ones align best with your aspirations and talents.

1.2 Developing Your Unique Look and Style

As a model, your appearance is a crucial aspect of your success. We will delve into the importance of taking care of your skin, hair, and overall physical well-being. Embracing a healthy lifestyle, maintaining a balanced diet, and incorporating exercise into your routine are essential for both your physical health and your ability to showcase your best self in front of the camera. Additionally, we will discuss the significance of cultivating your own sense of style and staying up-to-date with the latest fashion trends.

1.3 Posing and Body Language

The art of posing is a fundamental skill for any model. We will explore different posing techniques that enhance your body's natural lines and create visually appealing compositions. Understanding body language, facial expressions, and conveying emotions through your poses will set you apart as a versatile and expressive model. We will provide tips and exercises to help you develop confidence and grace in front of the camera.

1.4 Building Your Modeling Portfolio

A modeling portfolio is your visual resume and a crucial tool for showcasing your range and potential to potential clients and agencies. We will guide you through the process of building a compelling portfolio, including selecting the right photographs, collaborating with photographers, and curating a diverse collection of images that highlight your versatility as a model. We will also discuss the importance of regularly updating your portfolio to reflect your growth and evolving style.

1.5 Navigating the Industry: Agencies and Self-Promotion

Understanding the role of modeling agencies and how they can support your career is essential. We will explore the benefits of working with reputable agencies, including their network of industry connections, guidance, and access to professional opportunities. Additionally, we will discuss the importance of self-promotion, building your personal brand, and utilizing online platforms and social media to showcase your work and attract attention from potential clients.

By mastering the basics of modeling, you are setting yourself up for success in this dynamic and competitive industry. This chapter serves as a solid foundation, equipping you with the knowledge and skills necessary to pursue your modeling aspirations. As you navigate the diverse facets of modeling, remember that dedication, perseverance, and a commitment to continual growth are key. With a strong foundation and a passion for the craft, you are ready to embark on an exciting journey toward realizing your dreams as a model.

Chapter 2:
Preparing for a Modeling Career

In this chapter, we will discuss the steps you need to take to prepare for a modeling career. This includes developing a portfolio, finding an agent, and creating a personal brand. We will also cover the importance of maintaining a healthy lifestyle and taking care of your body.

Preparing for a modeling career requires a lot of hard work, dedication, and preparation. In this chapter, we will discuss the steps you need to take to prepare for a modeling career, including developing a portfolio, finding an agent, and creating a personal brand.

Congratulations on taking the first steps toward your modeling career! In this chapter, we will delve into the essential steps and preparations you need to undertake to set yourself up for success in the competitive world of modeling. From honing your skills to building a professional network, we will guide you through the process of preparing for a thriving modeling career.

2.1 Developing Confidence and Professionalism

Confidence and professionalism are the cornerstones of a successful modeling career. We will explore strategies to boost your self-confidence, including positive self-talk, visualization techniques, and embracing your unique qualities. Professionalism is equally important, and we will discuss the importance of punctuality, communication skills, and maintaining a positive attitude during photo shoots, casting calls, and runway shows. By cultivating these attributes, you will leave a lasting impression and build a reputation as a reliable and professional model.

2.2 Acquiring Modeling Skills and Techniques

As a model, it's essential to continuously develop and refine your skills. We will delve into the various techniques used in runway modeling, including posture, walking style, and choreography. Additionally, we will explore posing techniques for both photography and videography, including understanding camera angles, body awareness, and conveying emotions through your poses. By investing time and effort into practicing these skills, you will become a versatile and sought-after model.

2.3 Professional Photoshoots and Test Shoots

Professional photoshoots are an integral part of a model's career. We will guide you through the process of collaborating with photographers, stylists, and makeup artists to create stunning visuals that showcase your unique abilities and range. We will also discuss the importance of test shoots, which allow you to build your portfolio, experiment with different looks, and establish working relationships within the industry. Understanding the dynamics of a photoshoot and how to effectively communicate and collaborate with the team is key to achieving exceptional results.

2.4 Building a Professional Network

Building a strong professional network is crucial in

the modeling industry. We will explore different avenues for networking, including attending industry events, fashion shows, and casting calls. We will discuss the importance of making genuine connections with industry professionals, such as photographers, stylists, designers, and other models. Additionally, we will explore the power of online networking through social media platforms and industry-specific websites. By actively building relationships and fostering connections, you open doors to exciting opportunities and collaborations.

2.5 Education and Continuing Growth

Never stop learning and growing as a model. We will discuss the value of education and the importance of staying informed about the fashion industry, trends, and the evolving modeling landscape. Additionally, we will explore opportunities for further education, such as attending modeling workshops, fashion courses, and industry seminars. By investing in your ongoing development, you will remain relevant, adaptable, and equipped to excel in a rapidly changing industry.

Preparing for a modeling career is an exciting and transformative process. By focusing on developing confidence, professionalism, and honing your modeling skills, you will position yourself for success. Remember, preparation is key, and the journey towards a thriving modeling career requires dedication, perseverance, and a commitment to continual growth. In the next chapter, we will explore the world of casting calls and auditions, providing you with the knowledge and tools to make a memorable impression and secure coveted opportunities.

Developing a Portfolio:

A modeling portfolio is a collection of photographs that showcases your skills and abilities as a model. It is essential to have a strong portfolio to show to potential clients and agents. Your portfolio should include a variety of photographs that showcase your versatility as a model. This includes headshots, full-body shots, and action shots.

When developing your portfolio, it is important to work with a professional photographer who has experience in the fashion industry. They will be able to help you create a portfolio that showcases your strengths and highlights your unique qualities as a model.

Finding an Agent:

A modeling agent is a professional who represents models and helps them find work in the industry. They are responsible for finding modeling jobs, negotiating contracts, and managing your career. Finding the right agent is essential to your success as a model.

To find an agent, you can start by researching reputable modeling agencies in your area. Look for agencies that have a good reputation in the industry and have experience working with models in your category. You can also attend open calls or submit your portfolio to agencies online.

Creating a Personal Brand:

Creating a personal brand is essential to your success as a model. Your personal brand is how you present yourself to the world and how you differentiate yourself from other models. It includes your personality, style, and overall image.

To create a personal brand, you need to identify your unique qualities and strengths as a model. This includes your physical attributes, your personality, and your interests. You should also develop a signature style that sets you apart from other models.

It is also important to have a strong online presence. This includes having a professional website and social media accounts that showcase your portfolio and personal brand.

Maintaining a Healthy Lifestyle:

Maintaining a healthy lifestyle is essential to your success as a model. This includes eating a healthy diet, exercising regularly, and getting enough sleep. Models need to have a fit and toned physique, and it is essential to take care of your body to maintain your appearance.

Preparing for a modeling career requires a lot of hard work and dedication. It is essential to develop a strong portfolio, find the right agent, create a personal brand, and maintain a healthy lifestyle. With the right preparation and dedication, anyone can become a successful model.

Chapter 3:

The Runway

In this chapter, we will explore the world of runway modeling. We will cover the different types of runway shows, the skills you need to walk the runway, and the importance of professionalism and confidence. We will also discuss the challenges of runway modeling and how to overcome them.

The runway is one of the most exciting and glamorous aspects of modeling. It is where models get to showcase the latest fashion designs and walk in front of a live audience. In this chapter, we will explore the world of runway modeling, including the different types of runway shows, the skills you need to walk the runway, and the importance of professionalism and confidence.

Types of Runway Shows:

There are several different types of runway shows, each with its own unique style and requirements. The most common types of runway shows include:

1. Fashion Week Shows: These are the most prestigious and high-profile runway shows, featuring the latest fashion designs from top designers.

2. Ready-to-Wear Shows: These shows feature clothing that is ready to be worn and purchased by consumers.

3. Couture Shows: These shows feature high-end, custom-made clothing that is often one-of-a-kind.

Skills for Walking the Runway:

Walking the runway requires a combination of natural talent and learned skills. Some of the essential skills for walking the runway include:

1. Posture: Models need to have good posture and walk with confidence.

2. Stride: Models need to have a strong and confident stride, with their arms and legs moving in sync.

3. Timing: Models need to be able to time their movements with the music and the other models on the runway.

4. Facial Expressions: Models need to be able to convey different emotions with their facial expressions.

5. Professionalism: Models need to be professional and reliable, showing up on time and ready to work.

Called To Intercede Volume 13

Praying for Churches

Dr. Monique Rodgers

Importance of Professionalism and Confidence:

Professionalism and confidence are essential to success in the runway modeling industry. Models need to be able to work well with designers, stylists, and other industry professionals. They also need to be able to handle the pressure of performing in front of a live audience.

Confidence is also essential to success in the runway modeling industry. Models need to be able to walk with confidence and showcase the clothing with grace and poise. They also need to be able to handle any mishaps that may occur on the runway, such as a wardrobe malfunction or a stumble.

The runway is an exciting and glamorous aspect of

modeling. To succeed in the runway modeling industry, models need to have a combination of natural talent and learned skills. They also need to be professional, confident, and able to handle the pressure of performing in front of a live audience. With the right preparation and dedication, anyone can become a successful runway model.

Chapter 4:

Photo Shoots

In this chapter, we will discuss the art of modeling for photo shoots. We will cover the different types of photo shoots, the skills you need to pose for the camera, and the importance of communication with the photographer. We will also discuss the challenges of photo shoots and how to overcome them.

Photo shoots are an essential part of modeling. They are where models get to showcase their skills and abilities in front of the camera and create stunning images that will be used in advertisements, magazines, and other media. In this chapter, we will discuss the art of modeling for photo shoots, including the different types of photo shoots, the skills you need to pose for the camera, and the importance of communication with the photographer.

Types of Photo Shoots:

There are several different types of photo shoots, each with its own unique style and requirements. The most common types of photo shoots include:

1. Editorial Shoots: These shoots are used for fashion magazines and feature high-end clothing and accessories.

2. Commercial Shoots: These shoots are used for advertisements and catalogs and feature a variety of products and services.

3. Beauty Shoots: These shoots focus on hair and makeup and are used for beauty products and services.

Skills for Posing for the Camera:

Posing for the camera requires a combination of natural talent and learned skills. Some of the essential skills for posing for the camera include:

1. Body Positioning: Models need to know how to position their bodies to create the desired effect.

2. Facial Expressions: Models need to know how to convey different emotions with their facial expressions.

3. Movement: Models need to know how to move their bodies to create dynamic and interesting images.

4. Confidence: Models need to be confident in themselves and their abilities.

5. Professionalism: Models need to be professional and reliable, showing up on time and ready to work.

Importance of Communication with the Photographer:

Communication with the photographer is essential to success in photo shoots. Models need to be able to understand the photographer's vision and work with them to create the desired images. This includes discussing the concept of the shoot, the desired poses and expressions, and any other details that are important to the shoot.

Models also need to be able to take direction from the photographer and make adjustments to their poses and expressions as needed. This requires good communication skills and the ability to work well with others.

Praying for Churches

Dr. Monique Rodgers

Photo shoots are an essential part of modeling. To succeed in the photo shoot modeling industry, models need to have a combination of natural talent and learned skills. They also need to be able to communicate effectively with the photographer and work well with others. With the right preparation and dedication, anyone can become a successful photo shoot model.

Chapter 5:
The Business of Modeling

In this chapter, we will cover the business side of modeling. We will discuss contracts, negotiations, and the importance of understanding your worth as a model. We will also cover the importance of financial planning and building a sustainable career in the fashion industry.

Chapter 6:

The Future of Modeling

In this chapter, we will explore the future of modeling and the changes that are happening in the industry. We will discuss the impact of social media on modeling, the rise of diversity and inclusivity in fashion, and the importance of sustainability in the fashion industry.

The modeling industry is a complex and competitive business. To succeed as a model, it is essential to have a good understanding of the business side of modeling. In this chapter, we will discuss the different aspects of the business of modeling, including contracts, finances, and networking.

Contracts:

Contracts are an essential part of the modeling industry. They outline the terms and conditions of the modeling job, including the payment, the length of the job, and any other details that are important to the job. It is essential to read and understand the contract before signing it to ensure that you are comfortable with the terms and conditions.

It is also important to work with a reputable agent who can help you negotiate contracts and ensure that you are getting fair compensation for your work.

Finances:

Finances are an important aspect of the modeling industry. Models need to be able to manage their finances effectively to ensure that they are getting paid for their work and that they are able to support themselves financially.

It is important to keep track of your income and expenses and to set aside money for taxes and other expenses. It is also important to work with a reputable accountant who can help you manage your finances and ensure that you are in compliance with tax laws.

Networking:

Networking is an essential part of the modeling industry. Models need to be able to network effectively to build relationships with industry professionals and to find new job opportunities.

Networking can include attending industry events, reaching out to photographers and designers, and building relationships with other models and industry professionals. It is important to be professional and personable when networking and to always be prepared with a portfolio and business cards. The business of modeling is a complex and competitive industry. To succeed as a model, it is essential to have a good understanding of contracts, finances, and networking. It is also important to work with reputable agents and accountants who can help you navigate the business side of modeling. With the right preparation and dedication, anyone can become a successful model in the industry. Modeling is a challenging and rewarding profession that requires hard work, dedication, and a passion for fashion. In this book, we have provided you with the tools and knowledge you need to succeed in the industry. From the basics of modeling to the future of the industry, we hope this book has inspired you to pursue your dreams and become a successful model.

The modeling industry is constantly evolving, and the future of modeling is exciting and full of possibilities. In this chapter, we will discuss some of the trends and changes that are shaping the future of modeling, including diversity and inclusivity, the rise of social media, and the use of technology.

Diversity and Inclusivity:

Diversity and inclusivity are becoming increasingly important in the modeling industry. There is a growing demand for models of all shapes, sizes, and ethnicities, and the industry is starting to respond to this demand.

Many fashion brands and designers are now featuring more diverse models in their campaigns and runway shows, and there is a growing movement towards body positivity and inclusivity in the industry.

Praying for Churches

Dr. Monique Rodgers

The Rise of Social Media:

Social media is playing an increasingly important role in the modeling industry. Many models are now using social media platforms like Instagram and TikTok to build their personal brands and connect with fans and industry professionals.

Social media has also opened up new opportunities for models, with many brands and designers now using social media influencers to promote their products and services.

The Use of Technology:

Technology is also playing an increasingly important role in the modeling industry. Many brands and designers are now using virtual and augmented reality technology to create immersive and interactive experiences for their customers. There is also a growing trend towards using 3D scanning and printing technology to create custom-made clothing and accessories for models and customers.

The future of modeling is exciting and full of possibilities. With a growing focus on diversity and inclusivity, the rise of social media, and the use of technology, the modeling industry is evolving and adapting to meet the changing needs of consumers and industry professionals.

To succeed in the future of modeling, models will need to be adaptable, tech-savvy, and able to build strong personal brands. With the right preparation and dedication, anyone can become a successful model in the ever-evolving modeling industry.

Encouragement for Models

Being a model is not an easy job. It requires hard work, dedication, and perseverance. There will be times when you face rejection, criticism, and setbacks. However, with the right mindset and attitude, you can overcome these challenges and achieve your goals. In this chapter, we will discuss some motivational tips for models to help you stay focused and motivated on your journey.

Believe in Yourself:

The first step to success as a model is to believe in yourself. You need to have confidence in your abilities and believe that you have what it takes to succeed. Remember that every successful model started somewhere, and with hard work and dedication, you can achieve your goals.

Set Realistic Goals:

Setting realistic goals is essential to success as a model. You need to have a clear vision of what you want to achieve and set achievable goals that will help you get there. Break down your goals into smaller, manageable steps, and celebrate your achievements along the way.

Stay Positive:

Staying positive is essential to success as a model. You will face rejection and criticism along the way, but it is important to stay focused on your goals and maintain a positive attitude. Surround yourself with positive people who support and encourage you, and remember that every setback is an opportunity to learn and grow.

Take Care of Yourself:

Taking care of yourself is essential to success as a model. You need to maintain a healthy lifestyle, including eating a balanced diet, exercising regularly, and getting enough sleep. You also need to take care of your mental health, including managing stress and practicing self-care.

Stay Focused:

Staying focused is essential to success as a model. You need to stay focused on your goals and maintain a strong work ethic. This means being reliable, professional, and always striving to improve your skills and abilities.

Being a model is a challenging but rewarding career. With the right mindset and attitude, you can overcome any challenge and achieve your goals. Remember to believe in yourself, set realistic goals, stay positive, take care of yourself, and stay focused on your goals. With hard work and dedication, you can become a successful model and achieve your dreams.

Words of wisdom for models

As a model, you are embarking on a challenging and rewarding career. Here are some words of wisdom to help guide you on your journey:

1. Believe in yourself: Confidence is key in the modeling industry. Believe in your abilities and know that you have what it takes to succeed.

2. Stay true to yourself: Don't compromise your values or beliefs for the sake of your career. Stay true to who you are and what you stand for.

3. Be professional: Professionalism is essential in the modeling industry. Show up on time, be reliable, and always strive to improve your skills and abilities.

4. Embrace rejection: Rejection is a part of the modeling industry. Don't let it discourage you. Use it as an opportunity to learn and grow.

5. Take care of yourself: Your health and well-being are essential to your success as a model. Take care of yourself both physically and mentally.

6. Network: Networking is essential in the modeling

famous models of all time. She went on to become a successful businesswoman, author, and television personality.

2. Tyra Banks: Tyra Banks started her career as a model in the 1990s and went on to become one of the most successful models of all time. She later became a television personality, author, and businesswoman.

3. Iman: Iman started her career as a model in the 1970s and quickly became one of the most famous models of all time. She later became a successful businesswoman and philanthropist.

4. Kate Moss: Kate Moss started her career as a model in the 1990s and quickly became one of the most famous models of all time. She later became a fashion designer and businesswoman.

5. Gisele Bundchen: Gisele Bundchen started her career as a model in the 1990s and went on to become one of the most successful models of all time. She later became a philanthropist and environmental activist.

These are just a few examples of famous people who started their careers as models and went on to achieve great success in other fields. Their success shows that modeling can be a great starting point for a successful career in many different industries.

Modeling is a great career for many reasons. Here are a few:

1. Creativity: Modeling allows you to express your creativity and showcase your unique style and personality. You get to work with designers, photographers, and other creative professionals to create stunning images and fashion looks.

2. Flexibility: Modeling offers a lot of flexibility in terms of scheduling and location. You can work on a freelance basis and choose the jobs that fit your schedule and preferences.

3. Travel: Modeling often involves travel to different locations for photo shoots, fashion shows, and other events.

This can be a great opportunity to see the world and experience different cultures.

4. Networking: Modeling is a great way to build your professional network and make connections with industry professionals. This can open up new opportunities and help you grow your career.

5. Financial rewards: Modeling can be a lucrative career, with top models earning millions of dollars per year. Even for those just starting out, modeling can provide a good source of income and financial stability.

6. Personal growth: Modeling can be a great way to build your confidence, develop your communication skills, and learn how to work with others in a professional setting.

Overall, modeling is a great career for those who are creative, flexible, and willing to work hard. It offers a lot of opportunities for personal and professional growth, as well as financial rewards and the chance to travel and see the world.

Succeeding as a new model can be challenging, but with the right mindset and approach, it is possible. Here are some tips to help you succeed as a new model:

1. Build a strong portfolio: Your portfolio is your calling card as a model. It should showcase your best work and demonstrate your range and versatility as a model. Work with a reputable photographer to create a strong portfolio that will help you stand out.

2. Find a reputable agency: A good modeling agency can help you find work, negotiate contracts, and provide guidance and support as you navigate the industry. Do your research and find a reputable agency that has a good track record of success.

3. Network: Networking is essential in the modeling industry. Attend industry events, reach out to

photographers and designers, and build relationships with other models and industry professionals. Be professional and personable when networking and always be prepared with a portfolio and business cards.

4. Be professional: Professionalism is essential in the modeling industry. Show up on time, be reliable, and always strive to improve your skills and abilities. Be respectful of others and maintain a positive attitude, even in the face of rejection or criticism.

5. Stay in shape: Physical fitness is important in the modeling industry. Maintain a healthy diet and exercise regularly to stay in shape and maintain your appearance.

6. Be open to feedback: Feedback is essential to growth and improvement as a model. Be open to constructive criticism and use it as an opportunity to learn and grow.

7. Stay focused: Stay focused on your goals and maintain a strong work ethic. This means being reliable, professional, and always striving to improve your skills and abilities.

Overall, succeeding as a new model requires hard work, dedication, and perseverance. With the right mindset and approach, you can achieve your goals and become a successful model in the industry.

Praying for Churches

Dr. Monique Rodgers

100 Affirmations for Models

1. I am confident in my unique beauty and presence.

2. I embrace my flaws and consider them part of my unique appeal.

3. I am worthy of success and abundance in my modeling career.

4. I attract exciting and fulfilling modeling opportunities into my life.

5. I radiate confidence and grace on and off the runway.

6. I am grateful for my body and take care of it with love and respect.

7. I am a versatile and adaptable model, capable

of embodying various styles and looks.

8. I am deserving of recognition and appreciation for my hard work and talent.

9. I am a professional and reliable model, always delivering my best.

10. I attract positive and supportive individuals into my modeling journey.

11. I am constantly evolving and growing as a model and as an individual.

12. I am comfortable and at ease in front of the camera.

13. I trust my intuition to guide me in making the right career decisions.

14. I am grateful for every opportunity that comes my way, big or small.

15. I am a role model for aspiring models, inspiring them with my dedication and success.

16. I am confident in my ability to succeed in the competitive world of modeling.

17. I am comfortable expressing my unique personality and style through my work.

18. I am passionate about my craft and continually strive for excellence.

19. I am open to constructive criticism and use it to improve my skills.

20. I am proud of my accomplishments as a model and celebrate each milestone.

21. I am resilient and bounce back from setbacks with renewed determination.

22. I am surrounded by a supportive network of

industry professionals who believe in my talent.

23. I radiate positive energy and attract positive experiences into my modeling career.

24. I am a magnet for lucrative and fulfilling modeling contracts.

25. I am confident in my ability to handle any challenge that comes my way.

26. I am disciplined and committed to maintaining a healthy and fit lifestyle.

27. I am proud of my unique features and embrace them as assets in my modeling career.

28. I am constantly learning and growing, refining my skills as a model.

29. I am deserving of respect and fair treatment in the modeling industry.

30. I attract opportunities that align with my values and personal brand.

31. I am comfortable stepping out of my comfort zone to pursue new and exciting modeling ventures.

32. I am grateful for the supportive fans and followers who appreciate and admire my work.

33. I am a trendsetter, influencing the fashion industry with my style and presence.

34. I radiate beauty from within, and it shines through in all my work.

35. I am confident in my abilities and trust in the process of my modeling journey.

36. I attract photographers and creative teams who capture my essence beautifully.

37. I am focused and committed to my long-term modeling goals.

38. I embrace rejection as a stepping stone to success, knowing that each "no" brings me closer to a "yes."

39. I am a source of inspiration and empowerment to others through my modeling career.

40. I am grateful for the opportunities that allow me to travel and experience new cultures.

41. I have a powerful presence on the runway, captivating audiences with my grace and confidence.

42. I am deserving of fair compensation for my time, effort, and talent as a model.

43. I am grateful for the support of my loved ones, who cheer me on in my modeling journey.

44. I am a fierce competitor, always striving to improve and surpass my personal best.

45. I radiate professionalism in all my interactions, earning the respect of industry professionals.

46. I am proud of my unique heritage and use it to bring diversity and representation to the modeling industry.

47. I am open to collaborations that stretch my creative boundaries and showcase my versatility.

48. I am worthy of self-care and prioritize my physical and mental well-being.

49. I attract positive media attention that elevates my career and amplifies my message.

50. I am a trailblazer, breaking barriers and shattering stereotypes in the modeling industry.

51. I embrace challenges as opportunities for growth and personal development.

52. I am grateful for the lessons learned from both successes and failures in my modeling career.

53. I am a magnet for high-profile fashion campaigns and editorial features.

54. I am confident in expressing my opinions and advocating for positive changes in the modeling industry.

55. I radiate elegance and sophistication in all

aspects of my modeling career.

56. I attract collaborations with renowned designers who appreciate my unique style.

57. I am dedicated to continuously expanding my modeling skills through ongoing education and training.

58. I am a source of inspiration to young models, guiding them with kindness and wisdom.

59. I attract financial abundance through my modeling career, allowing me to live a comfortable and fulfilling life.

60. I am grateful for the experiences that allow me to connect with diverse cultures and communities.

61. I embrace opportunities for personal

branding and leverage my platform to make a positive impact.

62. I am confident in my abilities to succeed in any market or fashion capital worldwide.

63. I radiate positive energy during castings and auditions, leaving a lasting impression on casting directors.

64. I am deserving of equal opportunities and fair treatment in all aspects of my modeling career.

65. I am a trendsetter, influencing fashion and beauty standards with my unique style.

66. I attract reputable fashion publications that feature my work and showcase my talent.

67. I am grateful for the support and guidance of

mentors who have helped shape my modeling career.

68. I am comfortable stepping into various roles and personas, bringing versatility to my modeling portfolio.

69. I am a brand ambassador for products and causes I believe in, making a positive impact through my endorsements.

70. I radiate joy and enthusiasm, infusing every project I undertake with passion and creativity.

71. I am resilient in the face of rejection, using it as motivation to work harder and prove myself.

72. I attract positive collaborations with other talented individuals, creating memorable and impactful work.

73. I am grateful for the opportunities that allow me to use my modeling platform for philanthropic endeavors.

74. I am a source of inspiration to others, encouraging them to pursue their dreams fearlessly.

75. I radiate positivity and kindness, fostering a supportive and inclusive environment within the modeling industry.

76. I attract prestigious fashion events and shows that elevate my career and introduce me to influential industry professionals.

77. I am grateful for the experiences that allow me to embrace different cultures and celebrate diversity in the fashion industry.

78. I am confident in my ability to adapt to different fashion styles, trends, and creative visions.

79. I am deserving of praise and recognition for my contributions to the modeling industry.

80. I attract fulfilling collaborations that align with my values and allow me to express my true self.

81. I radiate professionalism in every aspect of my modeling career, earning the respect of clients and colleagues.

82. I am grateful for the opportunities that allow me to express my creativity and showcase my unique talents.

83. I am a magnet for prestigious fashion

designers who appreciate my professionalism and dedication.

84. I embrace opportunities to mentor and uplift aspiring models, sharing my knowledge and experiences with generosity.

85. I radiate beauty, elegance, and grace, captivating audiences with my presence.

86. I attract high-profile fashion campaigns that align with my personal values and ethics.

87. I am grateful for the support of my fans and followers, who inspire me to continue pushing the boundaries of my career.

88. I am a master of body language, exuding confidence and poise in every modeling assignment.

89. I am deserving of all the opportunities that come my way, and I embrace them with gratitude and enthusiasm.

90. I attract collaborations with renowned photographers who capture my essence and bring my vision to life.

91. I radiate authenticity, staying true to myself and my values in the midst of the fashion industry.

92. I am grateful for the opportunities that allow me to represent diversity and inclusivity in the modeling industry.

93. I embrace challenges as stepping stones to growth and breakthroughs in my modeling career.

94. I am a magnet for creative projects that push boundaries and redefine beauty standards.

95. I am deserving of respect and fair treatment in all my professional interactions as a model.

96. I attract inspiring and empowering opportunities that allow me to make a positive impact in the world.

97. I radiate confidence and charisma, captivating audiences and leaving a lasting impression.

98. I am grateful for the experiences that allow me to collaborate with talented artists and industry professionals.

99. I am a constant source of inspiration and motivation for myself and others in the

modeling industry.

100. I attract lucrative modeling contracts that bring financial stability and success into my life.

Remember to repeat these affirmations regularly, believe in them, and let them guide you towards a successful and fulfilling modeling career.

20 Tips for Fashion as models

1. Develop a versatile and adaptable personal style that showcases your unique personality while also being able to cater to different fashion genres and trends.

2. Prioritize comfort in your wardrobe choices, as feeling confident and at ease in your clothing will translate into more impactful photos and runway appearances.

3. Invest in a few essential wardrobe staples such as a well-fitted pair of jeans, a tailored blazer, a little black dress, and versatile footwear to create a foundation for various outfit combinations.

4. Pay attention to your posture and body language, as good posture enhances your overall presence and adds an air of confidence to your modeling.

5. Experiment with different hairstyles and makeup looks to discover what complements your features and brings out your natural beauty, while also being versatile for different fashion concepts.

6. Take care of your skin and maintain a healthy lifestyle to ensure a radiant complexion that will make you camera-ready and reduce the need for excessive editing.

7. Understand the importance of proper grooming, including maintaining well-groomed nails,

well-maintained hair, and overall cleanliness to present yourself professionally.

8. Develop a good understanding of different fabrics, textures, and how they drape on the body to enhance your posing and movement during photo shoots or runway presentations.

9. Practice walking confidently and gracefully in various types of footwear, as mastering the art of walking in heels and other shoes will be invaluable for runway shows and fashion events.

10. Pay attention to your body language during shoots and runway walks, as subtle movements and posing adjustments can make a significant difference in the overall impact of your photos.

11. Be open to direction and guidance from photographers and creative teams, as their expertise can help you create the desired visual story and bring out the best in your modeling.

12. Stay updated on current fashion trends and industry news to be aware of the latest styles, designers, and opportunities within the fashion world.

13. Network and build relationships with industry professionals, including photographers, stylists, makeup artists, and other models, as collaborations and connections can lead to exciting opportunities.

14. Embrace diversity and inclusivity in your modeling career by being open to working with

brands and projects that celebrate different body types, ethnicities, and cultures.

15. Practice posing in front of a mirror to become comfortable with different angles and expressions, allowing you to communicate various moods and concepts effortlessly.

16. Maintain a positive and professional attitude on set or during fashion events, as your behavior and attitude will leave a lasting impression on clients and collaborators.

17. Always be punctual and prepared for castings, shoots, and events, demonstrating your professionalism and respect for others' time.

18. Be open to constructive criticism and

feedback, as it can help you grow and improve as a model.

19. Take care of your overall health and well-being, including eating a balanced diet, staying hydrated, and engaging in regular exercise, as a healthy lifestyle will enhance your energy and radiance.

20. Remember to have fun and enjoy the journey. Modeling is an exciting and dynamic career, so embrace every opportunity to learn, grow, and express your creativity.

By implementing these fashion tips, you will be well on your way to building a successful and fulfilling modeling career.

About the Author

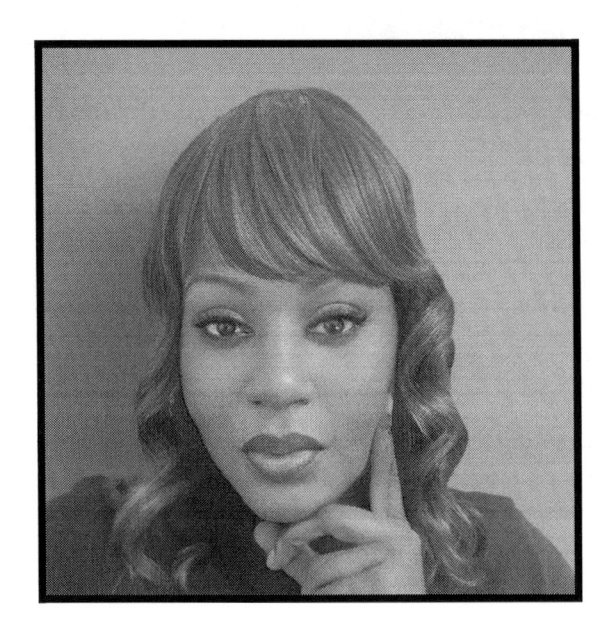

Dr. Monique Rodgers is an international bestselling author, CEO, visionary, master business coach, certified vegan health coach, motivational speaker, model, entrepreneur, educator, and literary genius. Dr. Rodgers excels today as a notable writing coach, founder, and serial entrepreneur. Throughout the course of her career, she has written such prolific works such as Hello! My name is Millennial. Picking up the Pieces, The Mystical

Called To Intercede Volume 13

Praying for Churches

Dr. Monique Rodgers

Land of Twinville, Falling in Love with Jesus, Accelerate, Overcoming Writer's Block, Just Breathe, Called to Intercede Volumes 1-13, I am Black History and many more. She has also been included as a co-author in collaborations such as Jumpstart Your Mind, Speak Up We Deserve to be Heard, Finding Joy in the Journey Volume 2, and Let the Kingdompreneurs Speak. Due to her outstanding breadth of experience, Dr. Rodgers has been featured on Rachel Speaks radio program, The Love Walk Podcast, The Glory Network, God's Glory Radio Show, The Miracle Zone, The Healing Zone, The Joyce Kiwani Adams Show, Coach Monique Ph.D. radio show, and many more. She has graced numerous platforms worldwide. She served as a TV host for WATCTV. She has been featured in Heart and Soul magazine, My Story the Magazine, and Kish Magazine's Top 20 Authors of 2021. She has also been featured in Marquis Who's Who in America

2021-2022. She also assisted in various volunteer work including an executive team member for Lady Deliverers Arise, Aniyah Space, and a board member for the I Am My Sister organization. She is also a certified master business coach, certified vegan health coach, and a health advocate. She has served in various leadership positions in business and in ministry. She is currently an Awakening Prayer hub leader for the city of Raleigh under the tutelage of Apostle Jennifer LeClaire. She is an ambassador for Kingdom Sniper Institute under the mentorship of Evangelist Latrice Ryan. As an expert in her field, Dr. Rodgers earned an undergraduate degree through Oral Roberts University as well as a Master of Science degree and a doctorate in global leadership through Colorado Technical University. She has also studied at The Black Business School online. Looking towards her future, Dr. Rodgers intends to expand upon her expertise and continue serving through ministry for God. She aspires to help over one hundred authors to complete and publish their books, help intercessors to draw closer to God and help train marketplace prophets and leaders for success.

Praying for Churches

Dr. Monique Rodgers

Contact information:

www.getwriteoncoaching.com

Facebook: www.facebook.com/moniquerodgers2

Instagram: @drroyalty7

Twitter: @DrMonique7

LinkedIn: Dr. Monique Rodgers

YouTube: Dr. Monique Rodgers

Clubhouse: @DrMonique7

Made in the USA
Middletown, DE
02 July 2023